Welcome to your Skills for Dementia Care Learning Resource

Introduction

Welcome to module 305 of the JPA Skills for Dementia Care Learning Resource. This resource will enable you to cascade your knowledge and understanding of individuals who may have specific needs for receiving medication because of their experience of dementia. Learners will develop their knowledge of these medication requirements.

Learning outcomes

On completion of module 305, you will have guided learners to meet the learning outcomes of the Qualifications and Credit Framework Dementia Unit 305.

Learners will:

1. Understand the common medications available to, and appropriate for, individuals with dementia.

2. Understand how to provide person-centred care to individuals with dementia through the appropriate and effective use of medication.

Preparation notes

*   To deliver this learning resource, you must be knowledgeable about the most up to date information in medication for individuals with dementia. Because this is constantly being researched and developed, it is recommended that you keep your knowledge up to date by using the Social Care Institute for Excellence (SCIE) free information and e-learning by visiting the Dementia Gateway at www.scie.org.uk/dementia. You will also find regular updates on the Alzheimer's Society web site at www.alzheimers.org.uk

*   There is a self-directed learning activity of approximately two hours' duration at the start of this module and you will send learners information on completing this, with their joining instructions. The purpose of this pre-workshop activity is to ensure that the most current information about medication is taught. **You should therefore also complete the self-directed learning activity before delivering this module.**

*   You must read through the entire trainer's guide, familiarising yourself thoroughly with its contents.

*   **The Skills for Dementia Care learner's workbook** contains fact sheets and exercises, asking learners to make links, write descriptions and discuss issues with you, so do check whether learners have literacy/numeracy difficulties. You may need to speak to their manager/supervisor to decide on any required steps to provide your learners with information in a different way.

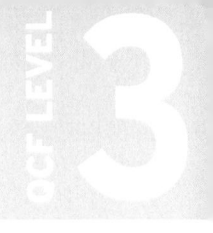

- The learner's workbook also includes a **learning record**, to show outcomes and the time spent in guided and self-directed learning. This workbook meets the learning outcomes and assessment criteria of the Qualifications and Credit Framework Dementia Unit 305. There is space for you to sign that learners have completed this module and for learners' QCF assessor to sign that the learners have achieved the required knowledge level.

- **The Skills for Dementia Care CD** contains the PowerPoint presentation which you will use during your training session. Before the start of the course, you should practise projecting the presentation, to ensure your familiarity with it.

- You will need to print the **confirmation letter** (on your CD) to give to each learner's manager/supervisor. This letter confirms that learners are undertaking module 305 training and indicates the amount of time required to complete the training sessions and work-based activities. It alerts the manager/supervisor to the need to provide ongoing support to each learner and to sign off each learner's learning diary, where indicated.

- You will also need to print the **joining instructions letter** (on your CD). This letter outlines information about the module. You should complete the relevant joining instructions and then send one to each learner, before the first attendance.

- Finally, you should print **certificates** and **evaluations sheets** (on your CD) to give to learners at the end of session 2.

To facilitate the training sessions, you will need:

- flip chart and pens.
- projector and/or laptop.
- PowerPoint presentation (on your CD)
- spare pens and paper for learners, if required.
- a learner's workbook for each learner.
- a certificate and evaluation sheet for each learner.
- You will find a notes box in this trainer's guide, at the end of each session. This is for your own personal use, to record ideas as you develop your skills in using this learning resource.

Confidentiality

Remind learners about the need, during training, to maintain the confidentiality of individuals, carers and others. State clearly that names should not be used and that all information shared during training must not be shared outside of sessions. Learners will need to show their workbook to their manager/supervisor. When asked to provide examples of service users, remind learners to refer to them as 'individual A' or 'Mr/Mrs/Miss A', rather than using any actual names.

Be mindful of any safeguarding issues which may emerge, following your agreed ways of working in addressing these.

Dementia can be a sensitive topic which may arouse deep feelings in carers, so a supportive atmosphere and respect for confidentiality are important. Where issues of concern (personal or work-related) arise during sessions, ensure that individuals are supported to take this up outside of sessions and that an agreement is reached about how to take any issue forward.

Timing

This module has a seven-hour programme of guided learning. This is presented in two sessions. You can choose whether to present the whole programme in one day or to split the programme into half days – or even shorter sessions on separate days.

This module has a further five hours of self-directed learning. There is a self-directed learning activity of approximately two hours' duration at the start of this module and you will have sent learners information on completing this, with their joining instructions. There is a further three hours of self-directed learning activity scheduled at the end of the module. You should agree, with learners and their manager/supervisor, when this will be completed. Explain that they should record in their learning record, the time spent and those activities carried out.

Hours of learning: On completion of module 305, learners will be able to provide evidence of the time taken to complete this course of study which meets the hours of learning criteria of the Qualifications and Credit Framework Dementia Unit 305.

To achieve the QCF credit of 2 points, learners will have completed:

- Seven hours' guided learning.
- Five hours' private study.
- Five hours' assessment with their QCF assessor.

Terminology

The content of this learning resource is written to be accessible and user-friendly. It is in keeping with the drive for personalised services and partnership approaches. The following terms are used:

individual	the person who is being supported/treated/cared for
work setting	the place where the individual is receiving support/treatment/care
agreed ways of working	policies/procedures/contracts/agreements
carer	partner/family/friends/neighbours
others	other professionals supporting/treating/caring for the individual

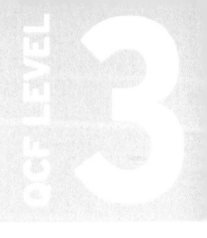

Assessment Criteria

On completion of module 305, learners will be able to provide evidence of knowledge which meets the assessment criteria of the Qualifications and Credit Framework Dementia Unit 305.

Learners will be able to:

1.1 Outline the most common medications used to treat symptoms of dementia.

1.2 Describe how commonly used medications affect individuals with dementia.

1.3 Explain the risks and benefits of anti-psychotic medication for individuals with dementia.

1.4 Explain the importance of recording and reporting side effects / adverse reactions to medication.

1.5 Describe how 'as required' (PRN) medication can be used to support individuals with dementia who may be in pain.

2.1 Describe person-centred ways of administering medicines whilst adhering to administration instructions.

2.2 Explain the importance of advocating for an individual with dementia who may be prescribed medication.

Content

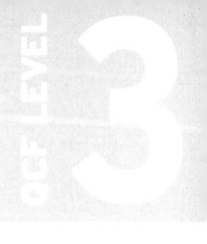

Session 1. Common medications available to, and appropriate for, individuals with dementia

Programme

30 minutes   Welcome and introduction to module 305

45 minutes   Session 1.1: The most common medications used to treat symptoms of dementia

45 minutes   Session 1.2: How commonly used medications affect individuals with dementia

15 minutes   Break

45 minutes   Session 1.3: The risks and benefits of anti-psychotic medication for individuals with dementia

45 minutes   Session 1.4: The importance of recording and reporting side effects / adverse reactions to medication

50 minutes   Session 1.5: How 'as required' (PRN) medication can be used to support individuals with dementia who may be in pain

NOTE: The timings of this programme are intended as a guide only. You should adapt timings according to discussions at the time and the level of prior knowledge among your group.

Welcome and introduction

Aim: To welcome and introduce learners to one another and to the learner's workbook.

Time: Allow 30 minutes.

Resources

Flip chart and pens

Projector and/or laptop

PowerPoint slide 1: Skills for Dementia Care – module 305: Understanding the administration of medication to individuals with dementia using a person-centred approach.

PowerPoint slides 2/3: Session 1 – Common medications available to, and appropriate for, individuals with dementia and learning objectives.

Learner's workbook pages 28/29

- **Show slide 1.** Welcome learners and introduce yourself.

- Provide information about domestic arrangements (fire exits, toilets, smokers' facilities).

- Check that learners have completed the self-directed learning activity in preparation for attending this session. Discuss with them, any difficulties they had with carrying out the activity and offer any additional support that may be needed. Explain to learners that they will be using their learning from the self-directed activity later in this session and you will all discuss this together then. If any learners have not completed the activity, advise them that they will be able to do so after the session.

- Give learners a learner's workbook or check that they have received one each, if these have been sent to them beforehand.

- Allow five minutes for learners to look through the workbook. Explain that information sheets are included, as well as activities for them to complete and space to write. Clarify that the emphasis is on shared practical learning, rather than formal teaching, based on the knowledge that we can all learn from one another. The success of the learning will depend, therefore, on everyone not only listening, but contributing as fully as possible to discussions.

- Refer learners to the learning record on workbook pages 28/29. Explain that this is a record of learning outcomes and time spent in both guided and self-directed learning. These meet the learning outcomes and the assessment criteria of the Qualifications and Credit Framework Dementia Unit 305.

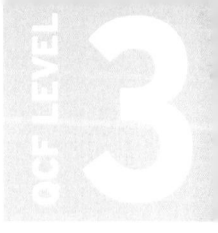

- Confirm that you will sign the learning record, when learners have completed this module. Explain that there is also space for their QCF assessor to sign that they have achieved the required knowledge level.

- Suggest that learners will need to keep the completed workbook for possible external inspection and for any future employment in the care sector.

- Explain that you have informed each of their managers/supervisors, by letter, that they are undertaking the learning programme.

- Acknowledge that dementia can be a sensitive topic which can arouse deep feelings in carers, so a supportive atmosphere and a respect for confidentiality are important.

- Explain that, where issues of concern (personal or work-related) arise during sessions, they will be taken up outside the sessions, with an agreement reached about how to take any issue forward.

- **Show slides 2/3:** Session 1 – Common medications available to, and appropriate for, individuals with dementia. Briefly outline the session's objectives.

Session 1.1: The most common medications used to treat symptoms of dementia

Aim: To enable learners to outline the most common medications used to treat symptoms of dementia.

Time: Allow 45 minutes.

Resources

Flip chart and pens
PowerPoint slide 4: Explaining the term 'dementia'
PowerPoint slide 5: Common cognitive symptoms associated with dementia
Learner's workbook pages 6-9

- **Show slide 4** and reinforce that the word 'dementia' is an umbrella term: a group name for the difficulties which individuals may experience when they have progressive diseases which affect the brain.

- Discuss with learners how the difficulties that an individual may experience can be a direct result of the changes to their brain, or be an indirect result of the impact of these changes on their relationships with others and on their emotional state.

- **Show slide 5** and discuss some of the common cognitive symptoms of dementia. Refer learners to **activity 1** on page 6 in their workbook and suggest to learners that they make notes as you discuss each symptom. Encourage them to contribute their experiences of the cognitive symptoms associated with dementia, possibly with individuals that they provide support to or with others. Ideas may include:

  - Memory loss: Unable to remember recent events, topics of conversation or names of individuals.

  - Planning and Sequencing difficulties: Unable to remember the steps needed to get dressed, make a meal or operate an appliance.

  - Speech and Language difficulties: Forgetting words or not understanding the words of others.

  - Problem solving difficulties: Unable to work something out.

  - Poor Judgement: Unable to weigh up the consequences of an action.

  - Disorientation in time, place and person: Unable to recognise where they are, what time or day it is, or who they are.

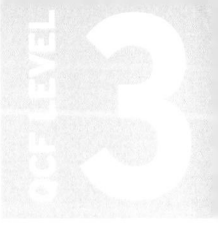

- Explain to learners that medication has an important role in supporting individuals to live well with dementia. Refer learners to **Information sheet 1** on page 7 and read through the first five paragraphs with them.

- Explain to learners that the terms drugs and medication are often used interchangeably. Medications are reviewed for their suitability by the government. In 2010 the government body responsible for reviewing medications is the National Institute for Clinical Excellence (NICE). Ask learners if they found any current information about the reviewing body when they carried out their pre-workshop self-directed learning activity. Discuss this information and add any information you have that is current about decisions concerning medication for individuals with dementia. Suggest that learners use the notes box on page 9 in their workbook to make a record of any current information.

- Ask learners to refer to the self-directed learning activity that they completed before attending this module and to call out the names of the medications that are used to treat dementia. Write all of these on the flip chart.

- Refer learners to **Information sheet 1** on page 7 in their workbook and read through the paragraphs headed **'Medications that work as acetylcholinesterase inhibitors.'** Identify from the flip chart list which of these medications are this type. These should include the following:

Trade name	Generic name
Aricept	Donepezil hydrochloride
Exelon	Rivastigmine
Reminyl	Galantamine

- Add the names of any of these that are not on the flip chart. There may be also be other medications as a result of new research and development and you should add these to the list. Allow learners time to copy the list into the notes box on page 7 in their workbook.

- Refer learners to **Information sheet 1** on page 8 in their workbook and read through the paragraphs headed **'Medications that work as glutamate blockers.'**

- Identify from the flip chart list which of these medications are this type. These should include the following:

Trade name	Generic name
Ebixa	Memantine

- Add the names of any of these that are not on the flip chart. There may be also be other medications as a result of new research and development and you should add these to the list. Allow learners time to copy the list into the notes box on page 8 in their workbook.

- Remind learners that in their self-directed learning activity, they noted the conditions that may be treated with each medication. Ask them to call these out and to record them in the relevant notes boxes on page 8 in their workbook. You will have researched and confirmed the most current information. Use the notes box below to record these in readiness for sharing this further information with learners.

Current information on conditions that may be treated with each medication:

- Remind learners to record the time spent in their self-directed learning activity on page 28 in their workbook.

- Reinforce the **KEY LEARNING POINTS:**

  - There are many different types of medication available to treat dementia, but a good assessment is necessary to ensure the right treatment is selected for each individual.

  - Not all medication treatments suit all types of dementia.

NOTES

This is for your personal use, to record your ideas as you develop your skills in using this learning resource.

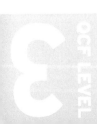

Session 1.2: How commonly used medications affect individuals with dementia

Aim: To enable learners to describe how commonly used medications affect individuals with dementia.

Time: Allow 45 minutes.

Resources

Flip chart and pens
PowerPoint slide 6: The benefits and risks of medication
Learner's workbook pages 10/11

- Remind learners of the types of medication described during session 1.1. The affects of these can be both positive and negative for the individual with dementia.

- Use two sheets of flip chart paper and write on one the heading 'benefits' and on the other, 'risks'. Ask learners to refer to the self-directed learning activity that they completed before attending this module and to call out the benefits and risks that they identified. Note these on the relevant flip chart paper and encourage discussion.

- **Show slide 6** to reinforce and add to the information on the flip chart lists. Refer learners to activity 2 on page 10 in their workbook and allow time for them to add the information from the flip chart and from the slide to the appropriate notes boxes.

- Refer learners to **activity 3** on page 11 in their workbook. Ask learners to get into three small groups. Allocate one discussion point to each group.

- Explain that each group should discuss their point by considering the advantages and disadvantages of using medication with these individuals and some of the challenges of ensuring that medication is taken appropriately. Suggest that they record their ideas in the relevant notes boxes and explain that they will be sharing their ideas with the rest of the group. Allow 15 minutes.

- Ask each group of learners to feed back their ideas and suggest that all learners record the ideas of others in the appropriate boxes on page 11 in their workbook. Some ideas are provided on page 16 of this guide to assist you.

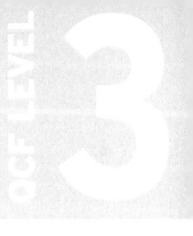

Discussion points for activity 3.

Individuals living in the community – alone in their own homes.
Advantages – the person can: remain at home; have a high quality of life; continue to carry out familiar activities; continue familiar social contact; be self-confident.
Disadvantages – side effects may go unnoticed; benefits difficult to monitor; benefits reported by the individual may not be actual; administration difficult to monitor; individual may forget to take medication or over-dose. The medication may be not be taken as prescribed.
Individuals living in the community – in their own homes with a family member.
Advantages - the person can: remain at home; have a high quality of life; continue to carry out familiar activities; continue family relationships and familiar social contact; be self-confident.
Disadvantages – the person may be reliant on the family member to monitor for side effects and benefits and to administer the medication. The medication may be not be given as prescribed.
Individuals living in residential homes.
Advantages – the person can: have a high quality of life; maintain independence; sustain social contact; be self-confident.
Disadvantages – the person may be reliant on untrained care workers, or who do not know the individual well, to monitor for side effects and benefits and to administer the medication. The medication may be not be given as prescribed.

- Discuss the importance of all care workers understanding the effect of commonly used medications on individuals with dementia.

- Reinforce the **KEY LEARNING POINTS:**

  - There are benefits and risks associated with medication for individuals with dementia.

  - There are different challenges for taking medication for individuals living in different situations.

NOTES

This is for your personal use, to record your ideas as you develop your skills in using this learning resource.

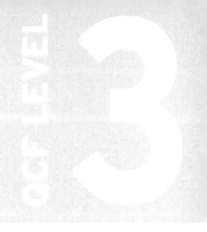

Session 1.3: The risks and benefits of anti-psychotic medication for individuals with dementia

Time: Allow 45 minutes.

Aim: To enable learners to explain the risks and benefits of anti-psychotic medication for individuals with dementia.

Resources

Flip chart and pens

PowerPoint slide 7: Common psychological and behavioural symptoms associated with dementia

PowerPoint Slide 8: Why is anti-psychotic medication used by individuals with dementia?

PowerPoint Slide 9: The risks of taking anti-psychotic medication.

Learner's workbook pages 12-14

- Refer learners to **activity 4** on page 12 in their workbook. Read through the first paragraph and discuss this information.

- **Show slide 7** and suggest to learners that they make notes as you discuss each of the common psychological and behavioural symptoms associated with dementia. Encourage them to contribute their experiences of these symptoms associated with dementia, possibly with individuals that they provide support to or with others. Ideas to assist you are provided in the table on page 19 of this guide.

- Reinforce that some of these symptoms may be a direct result of the condition causing the dementia, for example when a specific area of the brain has been damaged. For others the symptoms may be an indirect result of the impact of the experience of dementia on the individual's mental health and well-being.

Common psychological and behavioural symptoms associated with dementia.

Psychological	Behavioural
Depression Tearful, negative thoughts, loss of appetite, social withdrawal, suicidal, sleep disturbance	**Aggression** Physical or verbal attack.
Anxiety Bodily tension, repetitive questioning, agitation, over-eating, under-eating, sleep disturbance, obsessive/ compulsive behaviours.	**Agitation** Constant movement, restlessness, repetitive actions.
Psychosis Delusions (false beliefs or opinions), hallucinations (seeing or hearing something that may not be there), impaired insight, thought disorders, difficulty with social interaction.	**Pacing** Walking with no obvious sense of purpose other than to satisfy a drive for movement, may be unable to rest.
	Shouting out Repeatedly calling out.
	Sleep disturbance Sleep pattern that is unusual to the individual, unable to sleep, early morning waking.

- **Show slide 8** and refer learners to **activity 5** on page 13 in their workbook. Use the notes below and on page 20 to lead a discussion with learners about the benefits of anti-psychotic medication for individuals with dementia and why it might be used. Suggest that learners make notes in the relevant box in their workbook.

- **Reduction of distressing symptoms:** Behavioural and psychological symptoms such as aggression, agitation, delusions, depression and hallucinations are experienced by 80% of individuals with dementia. Anti-psychotic medication can improve an individual's emotional well-being.

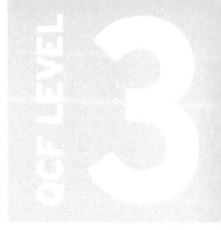

- **Supporting carers and others:** Carer burden is high when an individual with dementia has behavioural and psychological symptoms that carers find challenging. This often results in carers being unable to cope and becoming ill and the individual entering a care setting. Care workers and other service users in care settings can also be challenged by these symptoms, resulting in the individual becoming alienated and in possible staff absences and staff turnover.

- **Preventing care home or hospital admission:** There is evidence that anti-psychotic drugs have some modest treatment effect over short periods of time, particularly in reducing psychosis and aggression.

- **Show slide 9** and refer learners to page 13 in their workbook. Lead a discussion with learners about the risks of anti-psychotic medication for individuals with dementia. Explore how some of the side-effects of the medication may be assumed to be features of the individual's dementia and the risks associated with this. Suggest that learners make notes in the relevant box in their workbook.

- Refer learners to the list of anti-psychotic medication on page 13 in their workbook. Explain that some of these medications are rarely used and remind learners that new drugs are coming onto the market all the time and the list will change. They should use the notes box on page 14 in their workbook to add any new medications to this list.

- Remind the learners that the first line of treatment for behavioural and psychological symptoms experienced by individuals should be non-pharmacological therapies such as behavioural therapy, reminiscence therapy, validation therapy, exercise or multi-sensory therapy. Reinforce that anti-psychotic medication should be the last resort when all other methods have failed to alleviate the most distressing symptoms of dementia. If antipsychotic medication is to be used, careful monitoring and review must be implemented.

- Reinforce the **KEY LEARNING POINTS:**

  - Anti-psychotic medication should only be used as a last resort to manage the most distressing symptoms of dementia.

  - Careful assessment and monitoring should be implemented if anti-psychotic medication is to be used.

NOTES

This is for your personal use, to record your ideas as you develop your skills in using this learning resource.

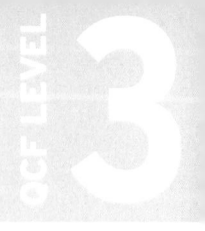

Session 1.4: The importance of recording and reporting side effects/adverse reactions to medication

Aim: To enable learners to explain the importance of recording and reporting side effects/adverse reactions to medication

Time: Allow 45 minutes.

Resources

Flip chart and pens
Learner's workbook pages 15/16

- Refer learners to **information sheet 2** on page 15 in their workbook. Read the first paragraph with learners and ask them if they can remember any of the side effects that have been mentioned in previous sessions. Refer to sessions 1.2 and 1.3 for examples.

- Ask learners to read through the remainder of information sheet 2 on page 15 in their workbook and to discuss this with a partner. Allow 20 minutes.

- Ask learners to share their ideas with the larger group and allow them time to make notes in the box at the top of page 16 in their workbooks.

- Refer learners to the reporting procedures outlined on page 16 in their workbook. Read through this with learners and ensure that everyone understands.

- If learners are already working in care settings, ask them to work in their small groups to consider the procedures there are in place for reporting adverse events and side effects. If they are unsure of these agreed ways of working, ask them to gather this information or ask their manger for this information, as a self-directed learning activity when they have completed this module.

- Refer learners to the notes box at the end of page 16 in their workbooks where they can record the agreed ways of working for reporting adverse events and side effects of medication. They can do this either in discussion in this activity or after the session as a self-directed learning activity.

- Reinforce the **KEY LEARNING POINTS:**
  - Administration of medication should be recorded according to regulations and agreed ways of working.
  - All side effects and adverse events should be recorded and reported to the relevant healthcare professional.

NOTES

This is for your personal use, to record your ideas as you develop your skills in using this learning resource.

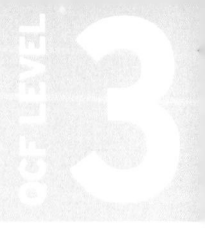

Session 1.5: How 'as required' (PRN) medication can be used to support individuals with dementia who may be in pain

Aim: To enable learners to describe how 'as required' (PRN) medication can be used to support individuals with dementia who may be in pain.

Time: Allow 50 minutes.

Resources

Flip chart and pens
PowerPoint slide 10: Pain management facts
PowerPoint Slide 11: Pain behaviours
Learner's workbook pages 17-19

- **Show slide 10** and refer learners to **activity 6** on page 17 in their workbook. Read through the points on the slide and allow time for learners to complete the facts in their workbook.

- Use the notes below to lead a discussion with learners about how pain relief is accessed by individuals with dementia. Suggest that learners record these in the notes box on page 17 in their workbook. Encourage learners to offer their own ideas and experiences. Issues will include:
  - How pain is recognised – the individual may express this is an unusual way and their behaviour may be mistaken for a symptom of their dementia.
  - How pain is assessed – the individual may be unable to indicate the location or the severity of their pain.
  - How pain relief is accessed – the individual's behaviour needs to be monitored as an indicator of the need for pain relief and their consumption of analgesics should be monitored.

- Reinforce that untreated pain can lead to behaviours that might be considered to be caused by the dementia process hence leading to incorrect treatment approaches. Ask learners to consider how they would know if an individual is in pain and to share their ideas.

- Refer learners to **activity 7** on page 18 in their workbook and read the first paragraph with them. **Show slide 11** and ask learners to work in pairs to match the pain behaviours listed on the slide, with the indicators in the right hand column of the table in their workbook. Allow 10 minutes.

- Discuss the correct responses with learners using this table:

Pain Behaviours	Indicators
Facial expressions	slight frown, sad, frightened face, grimacing, wrinkled forehead, closed or tightened eyes, any distorted expression, rapid blinking.
Changes in interpersonal interactions	aggressive, combative, resisting care, decreased social interactions, socially inappropriate, disruptive, withdrawn, verbally abusive.
Body movements	rigid, tense body posture, guarding, fidgeting, increased pacing, rocking, restricted movement, gait, or mobility changes.
Mental status changes	crying or tears, increased confusion, irritability, distress.
Verbalisations and Vocalisations	sighing, moaning, groaning, grunting, chanting, calling out, noisy breathing, asking for help.
Changes in activity patterns or routines	refusing food, appetite change, increase in rest periods or sleep, changes in rest pattern, sudden cessation of common routines, increased wandering.

- Explain to learners that there are a number of pain assessment tools that can be used to measure some of the indicators. A description of these is included on pages 18/19 in learner's workbooks.

- Reinforce the **KEY LEARNING POINTS:**

  - Good assessment of pain and the use of PRN analgesia can enhance the quality of life of individuals with dementia.

  - Observation and understanding of behaviours as indicators of pain is an important approach to supporting the well-being of individuals with dementia.

NOTES

This is for your personal use, to record your ideas as you develop your skills in using this learning resource.

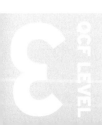
QCF LEVEL 3

Session 2. How to provide person-centred care to individuals with dementia through the appropriate and effective use of medication

Programme

15 minutes	**Summary of Session 1.**
45 minutes	**Session 2.1:** Person-centred ways of administering medicines whilst adhering to administration instructions
15 minutes	**Break**
50 minutes	**Session 2.2:** The importance of advocating for an individual with dementia who may be prescribed medication
20 minutes	**Preparing for a self-directed learning activity:** Investigating agreed ways of working
30 minutes	**End of module 305:** Recording learning

NOTE: The timings of this programme are intended as a guide only. You should adapt timings according to discussions at the time and the level of prior knowledge among your group.

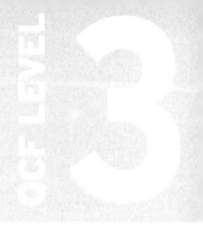

Summary of Session 1.

Aim: To allow learners to reflect on what has been learned from the previous session.

Time: Allow 15 minutes.

Resources

flip chart and pens

projector and/or laptop

PowerPoint slides 12/13: Understanding how to provide person-centred care to individuals with dementia through the appropriate and effective use of medication and learning objectives

PowerPoint slides 14/15: key learning points from session 1

- If you are leading this session on a separate date from session 1, refer to pages 9/10 of this guide to welcome learners back.

- **Show slides 12/13** and briefly outline the session's objectives.

- **Show slides 14/15** and summarise the key points that were covered during session 1.

- Ask learners to reflect on what they have learned during session 1 and use the flip chart to note key points learnt and areas for further development. Tell learners that you will be reflecting back on this list at the end of the module.

Session 2.1: Person-centred ways of administering medicines whilst adhering to administration instructions

Aim: To allow learners to describe person-centred ways of administering medicines whilst adhering to administration instructions.

Time: Allow 45 minutes.

Resources

Flip chart and pens
PowerPoint slide 16: The person-centred theory of dementia
PowerPoint slide 17: Person-centred actions
Learner's workbook pages 21/22

- **Show slide 16.** If learners have already explored this theory, briefly remind them of the factors. If this theory is new to learners, explain that understanding each of the factors and how they impact on an individual, is a helpful way of understanding the individual's experience of dementia.

- Refer learners to **activity 8** on page 21 in their workbook. Ask them to work in small groups to explore how each part of the model can be applied to understanding an individual's use of medication, by considering their own preferences. Allow 15 minutes.

- Ask learners to feed back their ideas and note them on the flip chart. Suggest that learners add the ideas of others to their notes. Some suggestions are provided on page 30 of this guide to assist you.

- **Show slide 17** and explain that the VIPS model was developed by Dawn Brooker as a method of applying person-centred theory to improve care services.

- Refer learners to **activity 9** on page 22 in their workbook. Ask learners to work in pairs and plan how they would apply the person-centred actions of the VIPS model to support Albert's medication needs, whilst adhering to any administration instructions that are required. Allow 20 minutes.

- While the group is carrying out the activity, prepare four flip chart sheets, each with a heading from the VIPS model.

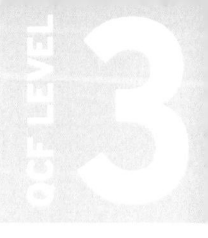

· Ask learners to feed back their ideas and note them on the appropriate flip chart sheet. Encourage discussion about each point. Suggest that learners add the ideas of others to their notes. Some suggestions are provided on page 31 of this guide to assist you.

Possible responses to activity 8.

Factor	Use of medication
Personality (Character and interests).	Does not agree with taking medication; believes you should 'work through' pain; believes taking medication is a sign of weakness; relies heavily on medication to address all needs; believes that medication is always the best.
Biography (Life history, skills and experience).	Religious beliefs affect which medications, or if medication is used; previous use of medication has affected willingness to use now; has always used natural remedies rather than prescription ones; has always investigated own needs.
Health (Physical ability and limitation. Mood).	Finds it difficult to read directions for use (visual difficulties); cannot take tablets and prefers liquids; cannot swallow large tablets; takes other medications and is careful of mixing them.
Neurological **S**tate (Cognitive ability and limitations).	When in pain, finds it difficult to read directions for use; has difficulty reading directions (English as a second language, dyslexia).
Social **P**sychology (Working with others).	Is reassured by hearing from others how medication has helped them; will only accept information about medication from a reliable source such as a GP or a Pharmacist; always discusses medication needs with partner/family member/friend.

Possible solutions to activity 9: How Albert can be supported using each of the person-centred actions of the VIPS model.

Valuing Albert
• Validating his feelings: showing that you understand he is distressed through the use of words and concerned facial expression and body language.   • Respecting his wishes and not trying to persuade him to take his medication while he is agitated.   • Supporting his dignity: not over-riding his wishes and enabling him to self-administer his medication if possible.

Individualised approach
• Using information about Albert's biography and personality to support him: enabling Albert to be in charge of taking his medication, checking what routine he had for taking his medication before he came to the home.   • Checking that the medication is in the format he is used to (tablets/solution).   • Involving Albert in planning a routine for taking his medication that fits with his wishes and with the prescription.

Albert's Perspective
• Understanding what triggers Albert's agitation and aiming to remove these triggers where possible (for example: a noisy environment, being rushed, being 'made' to do something).   • Understanding Albert's emotional needs: grieving for the loss of his wife and home, feeling a loss of control.

Social environment
• Reviewing the procedures in the home: have routines been established that do not take into account the need for a personalised approach.   • Ensuring care worker's communication skills are supporting Albert.   • Supporting care workers to view Albert as a unique individual, removing any labels of him as 'aggressive' which create an expectation and cause care workers to act negatively towards him.   • Monitoring that all care workers consistently apply the planned person-centred actions for supporting Albert.

- Reinforce the **KEY LEARNING POINT:**

  • Utilising a person-centred approach to administer medicines will facilitate and support the appropriate and effective use of medication for individuals with dementia.

NOTES

This is for your personal use, to record your ideas as you develop your skills in using this learning resource.

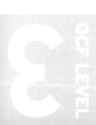

Session 2.2: The importance of advocating for an individual with dementia who may be prescribed medication

Aim: To enable learners to explain the importance of advocating for an individual with dementia who may be prescribed medication.

Time: Allow 50 minutes.

Resources

Flip chart and pens
PowerPoint slide 18: What is advocacy?
Learner's workbook pages 23/24

- **Show slide 18** and refer learners to **information sheet 3** on page 23 in their workbook. Read through the information and encourage discussion about each point. Suggest to learners that they make notes in the box provided at the bottom of page 23 in their workbook. Some discussion points to assist you are:

  - Who can be an advocate? Reinforce that this can be the individual speaking up for him or herself. Also refer to key principle number 4 and discuss if care workers can therefore be advocates, or does the advocate need to be independent of the service provider.

  - How does the information fit with legislation? Ask learners what legislation might be applicable. This should include mental capacity and safeguarding legislation.

  - For what aspects of care might an individual need an advocate's support? This should include any aspects that an individual wishes and might include advanced decisions eg. when an individual has specified particular types of treatment that they do not want should they lack the mental capacity to decide this for themselves in the future.

- Refer learners to **activity 10** on page 24 in their workbook. Ask the learners to divide into five groups and allocate one advocacy principle to each group. Ask them to consider the principle they have been given and identify how they can be an advocate for an individual who has been prescribed medication. Allow 10 minutes.

- Ask each group to feed back their ideas to the large group. Suggest that learners write these against each principle in their own workbooks. Some ideas are provided here to assist you.

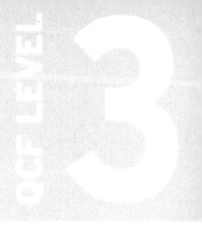

Principle 1.
Gather information about the medication wishes of the individual, using a range of methods of communication and checking for any written records such as an advance directive.
Be open and honest with the individual to establish a trusting relationship.
Be prepared to speak on behalf of the individual to express their views and wishes on their medication, even if they are in conflict with your own.

Principle 2.
Support the individual to make, or be involved in making, their own medication plan.
Support the individual to self-medicate if possible.
Review medication packaging and dispensers and enable the individual to manage these

Principle 3.
Provide the individual with all of the information they need about the benefits and risks of the medication, in a format and manner that they can understand.
Discuss the information with the individual and determine if they have understood by checking their responses.

Principle 4.
Remain loyal to the individual's best interests and express these even if they conflict with the agreed ways of working of the organisation.
Have support from managers and the organisation to be able to discuss freely and resolve any conflict of interests between the individual's wishes about their medication and the agreed ways of working.

Principle 5.
Offer the opportunity for individuals to have an independent advocate from outside of the organisation providing care.
Offer the choice of an individual advocate or group support – possibly through a service user association or with an advocacy group that is external to the care organisation.

- Reinforce the **KEY LEARNING POINT:**

  - It is important to offer an advocacy service for an individual with dementia who may be prescribed medication.

NOTES

This is for your personal use, to record your ideas as you develop your skills in using this learning resource.

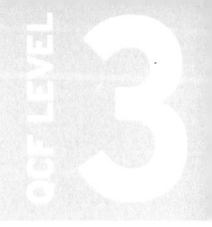

Preparing for a self-directed learning activity: Investigating agreed ways of working

Aim: To enable learners to become familiar with organisational policies, procedures and codes of practice for the administration of medication and for advocates.

Time: Allow 20 minutes.

Resources

Flipchart and pens

Learner's workbook pages 25/26 and 29

- Refer learners to **self-directed learning activity 11** on page 25 in their workbook. Explain that learners will complete this learning activity away from the workshop. It should take approximately three hours. Learners may discuss with their manager/supervisor how they take this time.

- Explain that the self-directed learning activity is an opportunity for learners to become familiar with organisational policies, procedures and codes of practice for the administration of medication and for advocates. If they are already working in a care setting, they should seek out the relevant documents. If these are not available, or they are not currently working in a care setting, learners can use the resources offered on page 25 in their workbook or they may search for others.

- Refer learners to the second part of the self-directed learning activity on page 26 in their workbook. Read through the instructions and ensure that everyone understands what they should do. Remind learners that they can discuss this activity with you or their manager/supervisor

- Suggest that learners record the source of their information in the notes box and share this information with their trainer and manager/supervisor.

- Remind learners to record the time taken in this activity in their learning record on page 29 in their workbook.

End of module 305: recording learning

Time: Allow 30 minutes.

Resources

PowerPoint slide 19 - key learning points from module 305
Learner's workbook pages 27-29
Evaluation sheets
Certificates

- **Show Slide 19** and reinforce the learning from this module. Refer to the flipchart of areas for further development compiled during the summary session at the beginning of session 2. Check with the learners that all areas have been covered and suggest ways of consolidating knowledge that might be missing.

- Refer learners to page 27 in their workbook and read through the information about completing the learning record on workbook pages 28/29. They should enter the time taken in total in guided learning. This will be approximately seven hours. Sign the appropriate boxes in the learning record and return them to the learners.

- Also explain that learners should enter the time taken in self-directed learning. This should be approximately five hours of private study and research. Learners should enter, in their learning record, those activities carried out. Arrange with learners that you, their manager or supervisor will sign the appropriate box in the learning record when they have completed the final self-directed learning activity after this course.

- On completion of this session, give out the evaluation forms and ask learners to complete them and return them to you.

- Give out certificates of attendance for this course. If your learners are undertaking a QCF qualification, you will need to arrange for a further certificate from the Awarding Organisation. This further certificate will be awarded when the QCF Assessor has signed the confirmation in the learning record, that assessment has taken place

- Thank learners for attending module 305 and inform them that there are further modules for dementia care in this JPA Skills for Dementia Care series:

NOTES

This is for your personal use, to record your ideas as you develop your skills in using this learning resource.

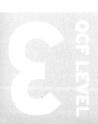